Health of Nation
Ambassador Dr Tom Mboya Okeyo

Part 1. Introducing the Health of Nation

Chapter 1. Definition of Health

The World Health Organization, which is the United Nations specialized agency for health matters defines health as "a state of complete physical, mental and social well-being and not merely the absence of disease or infirmity".

Access to quality health care encompasses a broader social, economic and political concept. It underscores a belief that improving health of the worlds peoples is an important measure of development.

Money spent for increased access to quality health care is considered a better investment in sustainable development. Development without significant investment in health care may not be sustainable.   Human beings will appreciate and enjoy other development initiatives such as improved infrastructure and elements of increased economic growth when they are in good health. It is therefore preferable that adequate investments aimed at improving health of the people precedes or is done concurrently with investments for other development initiatives.

Access to quality health care includes access to disease prevention, control and treatment services, including but not limited to access to affordable safe and efficacious health products. Health products includes medicines, vaccines and diagnostics.

Access to quality health care requires that the health professional providing the health service is registered and regulated under the relevant laws governing their practice and that the services being provided meet quality and safety standards as prescribed by the department responsible for health in the State or Country.

Chapter 2. Measuring health status of people

Considered together, observed trends of maternal mortality ratio together with neonatal mortality rate and under-five child mortality rate is useful for assessing the overall health status of people living in a state or country. This set of mortality experience can also provide useful information to guide further research on causes including identifying appropriate interventions required to improve the health status of people living in a given setting.

The World Health Organization Constitution contains a list of twenty-two functions. Two of these functions are to act as the directing and co-ordinating authority on international health work, and to establish and revise as necessary international nomenclatures of diseases, causes of death, and of public health practices.

In this regard, the World Health Organization publish the World Health Statistics. This publication contains useful information on maternal mortality ratio, neonatal mortality rate and under-five mortality rate for each Member State including estimates for all the six WHO Regions.

This set of mortality experience reported by State and by WHO Region considered together with other relevant research findings is useful for monitoring the overall health status of the worlds peoples. The World Health Statistics also contains additional information on other health matters of States.

If maternal, newborn and child mortality rates are declining but below the agreed target expectations, there is need to raise concern early enough and undertake research to identify possible causes, taking necessary corrective measures to get them back on track, right away. Where expectations or targets have been missed, there is an even stronger case to invest in research in order to inform further interventions and actions, as appropriate.

The global Maternal Mortality Ratio was reduced from 385 in 1990 to 216 in 2015, far below the expected target. Expected target reduction was 75% against the achieved reduction of 44%. Child mortality reductions were also below the expected two thirds reduction targets. Global neonatal mortality rate was reduced from 36 to 19 while the under-five mortality rate was reduced from 91 to 43 between 1990 and 2015.

Maternal, newborn and child health in a Nation State, if getting better by declining is a sign that the overall health status of the people living in that State is getting better, although there could be significant differences among communities living within the same State.

In 1990, the Infant mortality rate for Kenya was estimated to be 66 per 1000 live births, but was 54 per 1000 live births for Nyeri district and 220 per 1000 live births for South Nyanza district, both districts within Kenya.

Kenya is implementing one of the most comprehensive and revolutionary social, economic and political reforms in the world in order to reduce such inequalities within a country.

The Constitution of Kenya 2010, the only known Constitution of a State in the world which fully integrates the United Nations Bill of Human Rights, aims to progressively reduce inequalities within the State and provide access to quality health care for all Kenyans.

It is a decisive expression that access to quality health care and improving health status require social, economic and political reforms.

The people of Kenya wrote in the preamble of the Constitution of Kenya 2010 " We, the people of Kenya- Acknowledging the supremacy of the Almighty God of all creation: Honouring those who heroically struggled to bring freedom and justice to our land: Proud of our ethnic, cultural and religious diversity, and determined to live in peace and unity as one indivisible sovereign nation: Respectful of the environment, which is our heritage, and determined to sustain it for the benefit of future generations: Committed to nurturing and protecting the well-being of the individual, the family, communities, and the nation: Recognising the aspirations of all Kenyans for a government based on the essential values of human rights, equality, freedom, democracy, social justice and the rule of law: Exercising our sovereign and inalienable right to determine the form of governance of our country and having participated fully in the making of this Constitution: Adopt, Enact and give this Constitution to ourselves and to our future generations. God bless Kenya."

Chapter 3. Health status of worlds peoples by 2016

Based on information from the World Health Statistics 2015, and the United Nations General Assembly Resolution on Transforming our worlds: the 2030 Agenda for Sustainable Development of 2015, the global target to reduce maternal mortality ratio by three quarters between 1990 and 2015 was not met. The global target to reduce under-five mortality rate by two thirds between 1990 and 2015 was also not met. The proportion of deaths of children under-five years of age that occurred in the neonatal period increased significantly.

Although there was significant progress made, the targets were not only not met by end of 2015 but were considered off-track. Some of the other targets for the millennium development goals were either met or if not met progress appeared to be on-track. The observation that a significant number of countries were able to achieve national MDG targets for maternal mortality ratio and under-five child mortality rate, suggests that meeting the targets was doable.

The overall health status of the worlds peoples would have been better had the targets been met or surpassed. The results are a bitter pill to swallow by all leaders and peoples globally. It calls for redoubling of our collective commitment to the full realization of all the Millennium Development Goals, including the off-track Millennium Development Goals on maternal, newborn and child health. It is necessary that the new agenda of sustainable development goals builds on the Millennium Development Goals and completes all that which was not achieved as soon as possible.

It is a pointer to a significant problem which may be partly associated with inadequate investments in health and inadequate focus and commitment to universal health coverage among others. It is necessary to learn from States who were able to meet the maternal mortality ratio and under-five mortality rate targets of the millennium development goals. Improving the overall health status of the worlds peoples would benefit from continuous exchange of best practices.

That after 25 years of hard work, the global maternal, neonatal and child mortality and to some extent reproductive health targets are off-track as confirmed by research, calls for better decisive actions by all leaders.

Chapter 4. Fiscal stimulus package for maternal and child health

When in 2009, the world was confronted with the worst financial and economic crisis since the Great Depression, partly due to failures in financial regulation, supervision and monitoring of the financial sector, and inadequate surveillance and early warning, excessive risk-taking among others, world leaders took prompt and decisive actions by providing fiscal stimulus packages to affected financial institutions in order to get them back on track to profitability.

The underlying logic was that saving some of the affected financial institutions was for the greater good of the worlds peoples. The crisis was contained and there is improved global resilience.

If we could bailout global financial Institutions and get them back on track to profitability, surely we can bail out our loving women from deaths associated with pregnancy and child birth as well as our innocent children by ensuring that Maternal Mortality Ratio, Neonatal Mortality Rate and Under-five Mortality Rate targets are put back on tract to exceed target expectations of the new sustainable development goals before the year 2030.

The new agenda on the sustainable development goals promises "to promote physical and mental health and well-being, and to extend life expectancy for all, we must achieve universal health coverage and access to quality health care. No one must be left behind. We commit to accelerating the progress made to date in reducing newborn, child and maternal mortality by ending all such preventable deaths before 2030. We are committed to ensuring universal access to sexual and reproductive health-care services, including for family planning, information and education. We will equally accelerate the pace of progress made in fighting malaria, HIV/AIDS, tuberculosis, hepatitis, Ebola and other communicable diseases and epidemics, including by addressing growing anti-microbial resistance and the problem of unattended diseases affecting developing countries. We are committed to the prevention and treatment of non-communicable diseases, including behavioral, developmental and neurological disorders, which constitute a major challenge for sustainable development."

Basic to the happiness, harmonious relations and security of all peoples is health. The achievement of any State in the promotion and protection of health is of value to all human beings living or expected to be living on earth and in Space. Unequal development in different countries in the promotion of health and control of disease, especially communicable disease, is a common danger. If there is one area all human beings should work collectively to improve, it is health of the worlds peoples. The spirit that tuberculosis, Ebola, HIV, Influenza among other communicable diseases are a danger to all globally must be of serious concern to everyone, wherever they are living.

Chapter 5. Research and scale-up what works is the best option

Research needs to be undertaken to find possible causes for the inadequate progress towards improving the health of the worlds peoples after 25 years of hard work. Research findings should inform further interventions and actions.

These interventions would then be considered evidenced-based, cost-effective because they will be based on new research findings, and not on a "business as usual" approach.

There is need for all States to re-think investment in research as the top priority activity guiding implementation of interventions for achieving sustainable development goals 2030.

The Inter-agency task team on science, technology and innovation should prioritize research as the vehicle for guiding appropriate interventions for achieving health and health-related targets. Meetings of The High-Level Political Forum may consider giving high priority to reporting on progress of evidence for continuous improvement of health results for women and children in order to avoid being confronted with a repeat of inadequate progress in 2030.

Through research, it was discovered that the most effective weapon against tuberculosis is better housing, and increased access and appropriate use of anti-tuberculosis drugs. Research also shows that if we eradicate mosquitos responsible for transmitting the malaria parasite, and increase access to malaria diagnosis and treatment, including vaccines when available, malaria can be eradicated.

Therefore, for malaria we must declare a global war against mosquitos and all significant impediments to access to medicines and other health products required for the treatment of malaria, especially in the malaria endemic countries.

This requires States and and non-State actors to empower individuals at all stages of their life cycle, as appropriate to eliminate mosquitos and seek early treatment for malaria. Motivated health professionals are a critical success factor.

With regard to tuberculosis, all States must accord high priority to affordable housing for all citizens, including refugees and other migrant people as well as increased access to medicines and other health products for the diagnosis and treatment of tuberculosis. Ensuring access for all to adequate, safe and affordable housing and basic services, including upgrade of slums prevents the spread of tuberculosis.

The role of health professionals to deliver effective diagnosis and treatment is again paramount, and the critical success factor.

The International Centre for Insect Physiology and Ecology (ICIPE) together with the United Nations Habitat, both institutions with their headquarters based in Nairobi, Kenya, where the Headquarters of the United Nations Environmental Programme is based, consider being more effective in the alliance of States and United Nations specialized agencies, international organizations, scientific and professional groups and non-State actors in the fight against malaria and tuberculosis.

Building effective and efficient global partnership and adequate funding now is as important as the end of malaria and tuberculosis. We are all in this together.

Recognition of the supremacy of the Almighty God enables individuals to experience the universal connection of the natural law that governs all human beings irrespective of ethnic, cultural and religious diversity. The continuous pursuit of quality life, liberty and happiness is endowed by God, the Creator in all human beings, irrespective of one's social, economic, and political status in the world.

All leaders should strive to secure access to quality health care for all the worlds peoples. It is essential that Leaders are influenced through education and effective advocacy to demonstrate greater commitment to nurturing and protecting the health and well-being of the individual,

the family, communities and Nations. Good health is everything to me,
to you, to her, to him, to them and to us, all human beings.

Chapter 6. Involving and co-ordinating key-stakeholders

Managing relations between health and environment, education, cultural
beliefs and practices, religious beliefs, communication, energy,
disarmament, migration, human rights, peace and security, international
trade and other determinants of health impact on the efficiency and
effectiveness of re-engineering health governance to meet the
challenges of the 21st Century and beyond.   The World Health
Organization may consider exploring more effective mechanisms to
strengthen existing agreements with the United Nations, ILO, FAO,
UNESCO, International Atomic Energy Agency IAEA, International Fund
for Agriculture FAO, United Nations Industrial Development Organization
UNIDO, Universal Postal Union UPU, Office International des   pizooties in
order to improve the efficiency and effectiveness of cooperation in
implementing interventions for achieving health and health-relate tarets
of the sustainable development goals 2030.

However, careful attention be considered to avoiding as much as
possible getting the World Health Organization boxed into areas not
within its competency and mandate.

Governments have a responsibility for the health of their peoples which
can be fulfilled only by the provision of adequate health and social
measures. This responsibility for the health of the people of a State
requires effective leadership through regular reviews of national health
policies, health and health-related legislation, standards, guidelines,
research and monitoring.

The World Health Organization can be an effective partner in providing
technical assistance to Government on health matters, upon request.

Building on the significant progress the World Health Organization has
made on programmatic reforms, there may be need to review relevant
World Health Assembly Resolutions including ongoing programmatic
activities and partnerships which are related to achieving the health and
health-related sustainable development goals.

This may improve the quality of technical assistance required and
provide better focused scale-up technical assistance to Member States

in need. It may also contribute to better use of available human and financial resources.

Improving health of the worlds peoples is what pastes and holds the integrated nature of the sustainable development goals together as well as the interlinkages between them.

High priority needs to be accorded to strengthening technical and financial capacity of the Office of the WHO Country Representative in order to provide adequate technical assistance to State departments responsible for health, labour, security, economy, and finance to undertake comprehensive reviews of national health policy, legislation, strategy, standards and guidelines, and financing plans.

The aim should be to substantially increase domestic and international resources for financing implementation of interventions in order to achieve health and health-related targets of the Sustainable Development Goals 2030.

This proposed approach is based on previous experience at Country level when an effective and efficient Kenya WHO Country Office worked in partnership with the World Bank, United States Government agencies, United Kingdom Department for International Development, the German Government Development Agency KfW, UNDP, UNICEF among others to provide requested technical assistance to two joint national Committees and Secretariat composed of officers seconded from national departments responsible for health, security, economy and labour; the business sector; scientific and professional groups, and religious organizations develop and finalize Parliamentary Sessional Paper No 4 of 1997 on HIV///AIDS in Kenya and Parliamentary Sessional Paper No 2 of 2004 on National Social Health Insurance.

I had the privilege and honor to lead the Secretariat and provide public health policy guidance in the development of the two National Policy Sessional Papers. The implementation of Sessional Paper on HIV/AIDS in Kenya, which is still ongoing contributed to reduced adult HIV prevalence in Kenya from 14% to 6% between 1997 and 2007. The implementation of the Sessional Paper on National Social Health Insurance, which is also still ongoing contributed to increased universal health coverage in Kenya from 10% to 30% between 2005 and 2015. An estimated US$ 3 billion additional funding was mobilized from domestic and international development agencies for financing the two national health policy initiatives and related health activities.

We learned valuable new knowledge and experience on the critical role the people, their Parliamentary representatives, the business sector, religious organizations, senior public officials, and departments responsible for finance and security, as well as the the United Nations system and international development agencies contribute to the success or failure of national health policy making. This knowledge was hardly taught in the post-graduate schools of public health then.

Some of the secrets to success in managing national health policy development or review is for the Secretariat team to have timely and adequate knowledge and experience on the issue, if necessary take additional courses, participate in relevant international conferences and establish good networks with international think-tanks or caucuses of interest groups, if possible hold at least two national consultative conferences, be assured of access to quality technical assistance, have in place motivated multidisciplinary technical team with a wide range of expertise and knowledge of national policy procedures, adequate resources for operations and advocacy, be able to hold regular briefing of the Parliamentary Committee responsible for health matters, organize study tours and brainstorming sessions away from the Capital City when necessary, have excellent ability to communicate and write readily publishable materials for print and electronic media, have a media kit on key issues, stay away from the front-line, regularly brief the Minister or Cabinet Secretary and work towards getting the policy agenda to be an agenda of the Head of State and Government, with the Minister or Cabinet Secretary leading its implementation.

National health policy making is not a smooth process as there are strong competing interests among key stakeholders to be managed. We found it useful to keep key stakeholders close, informed as appropriate, participating, listening more, talking less, and keeping focus on the greater national policy goals. Ensuring that technical assistance provided is evidence-based, culturally sensitive, cost-effective, realistic and feasible in the country settings, is beneficial to all. The spirit of joint ownership and inclusiveness in policy dialogue helped to mobilize additional resources and strong commitment in implementation. Government, the United Nations system, Universities, professional groups, private sector, religious organizations, civil society and other actors working together to produce a negotiated implementable policy framework is slow but assures achieving sustainable solutions and improved coordination and better implementation efficiency and effectiveness.

The World Bank is very effective at bringing international development agencies onboard with additional co-financing or parallel financing arrangements around a new project during the project development stage and committing government to provide additional counterpart funding thus substantially increasing domestic resources. Parallel co-financing targeted towards activities implemented by non-State actors adds value to the overall national response around the negotiated policy framework.

Chapter 7. Right to health

In the Health of Nation, we also call for progressive implementation of the Right to health. The Office of the United Nations High Commissioner for Human Rights and the World Health Organization as part of commemoration of the 60th anniversary of the Universal declaration of Human Rights and establishment of the World Health Organization stated that the right to health is an inclusive right.

The right to health includes access to healthcare, safe drinking water and adequate sanitation, safe food, adequate nutrition and housing, healthy working and environmental conditions, health-related education and information as well as gender equality.

The right to health contains freedoms to be free from non-consensual medical treatment as well as from torture and other cruel, inhuman or degrading treatment or punishment.

The right to health contains entitlements. These include access to essential medicines, prevention, treatment and control of diseases, maternal, child and reproductive health, equal and timely access to basic health services, provision of health-related education and information, participation of the population in health-related decision-making at the national and community levels as well as a system of health protection providing equality of opportunity for everyone to enjoy the highest attainable level of health.

Non-discrimination, all services, goods and facilities available, accessible, acceptable and of good quality encompass right to health.

The United Nations International Covenant on Economic, Social and Cultural Rights as well as International human rights treaty bodies, and more than 100 National Constitutions recognize the right to health.

Chapter 8. Enabling non-State actors bridge the gaps

Monitoring the implementation of the right to health is a priority area for WHO leadership in consultation and cooperation with Member States, the United Nations, United Nations specialized agencies and other international organizations.

Progressive steps to achieving right to health also requires a strong WHO leadership team and effective coordination of other players in the global health arena, especially public private partnerships as well as other non-State actors. Public private partnerships have demonstrable ability to bridge the financing gaps in the fight against HIV/AIDS, Tuberculosis, Malaria as well as disease prevention through immunization. But they do face unique challenges.

During my work in global health, I came face to face with a significant number of these challenges affecting public private partnerships, non-state actors, UN specialized agencies and international organizations.

One morning in the year 2011 in Geneva, while serving as Ambassador Extraordinary and Plenipotentiary and Permanent Representative of the Republic of Kenya to the United Nations at Geneva, Conference on Disarmament and the World Trade Organization, I paid a courtesy call on the Executive Director of the GAVI Alliance.

The Executive Director looked worried and disturbed before requesting my Office to assist with finding a solution to enable UNICEF procure for GAVI Alliance, a new pneumococcal vaccine at an affordable price. The price lower than the one offered by manufacturers of the new pneumococcal vaccine to Pan American Health Organization (PAHO), the WHO Regional Office for the Americas.

Manufacturers of the new pneumococcal vaccine had committed to PAHO through a legally binding contract that should the manufacturers sale the vaccine to any other entity at a price lower than the price offered to PAHO, the lower price would be applied to PAHO retrospectively,

The Manufacturers of the new pneumococcal vaccine had decided that their business with PAHO was profitable, and as such declined to offer UNICEF the vaccine at the GAVI Alliance price, which was lower than the one offered to PAHO and more affordable.

That meant no new pneumococcal vaccines for GAVI supported countries, who also happened to have the most vulnerable health systems, globally.

Consultative meeting with the WHO Director-General on the same issue further highlighted how complex the matter was. The action taken by PAHO to have more value for money in the procurement of the new pneumococcal vaccine, which was legal within the terms of the contract, would effectively block implementation of differential pricing with regard to the GAVI Alliance. WHO promotes differential pricing in order to increase access to medicines and vaccines.

Further meetings with a representative of vaccine manufactures clarified that the Industry would supply the new pneumococcal vaccines at the GAVI price only if PAHO did not invoke the provisions in their procurement contract.

In order to resolve this problem, it became apparent that a combined diplomatic and political initiative was necessary. The then Kenyan Minister for Public Health and Sanitation together with colleagues from the African Region held informal discussions with a number of Ministers from PAHO and other WHO regions. A cascade of diplomatic and political engagements followed leading to the availability of the new pneumococcal vaccines in GAVI Alliance supported developing countries.

In Nairobi, Kenya, the President of the Republic of Kenya accompanied by senior officials from the GAVI Alliance from Geneva, Switzerland launched national immunization of children with the new pneumococcal vaccine in a colorful ceremony at the Kenyatta International Conference Centre.

Millions of preventable deaths and ill-health which would have been associated with pneumococcal pneumonia in children were prevented in GAVI supported countries.

This is one example, among many other diplomatic and political interventions we experienced during the World Health Assembly, and during other High-Level meetings of United Nations specialized agencies, the World Trade Organization, and Conference on Disarmament.

GAVI Alliance is a partnership of public and private sector to improve child health in the poorest countries by extending the reach and quality of immunization coverage within strengthened health services. It has a

Board which includes UNICEF, WHO, non-State actors, donor and
implementing country governments, vaccine industry representatives,
the Bill and Melinda Gates Foundation among others. The GAVI Fund is
administered by a Secretariat headed by the Executive Director.

Chapter 9. International Trade needs effective International Health Regulations

Disease outbreaks have adverse effects on international trade.
Improved health status of the worlds peoples including more effective
and efficient implementation of International Health Regulations to
prevent and control the spread of diseases is beneficial for the smooth
flow of international trade. The motivation in the 19th century for an
international health agency to promote cooperation among states on
health matters was Trade. International covenant on cholera was
among the first negotiated international treaties of the 19th Century
under the auspices of the International Sanitary Conference.

Trade policies affect public health policy. Trade can create wealth
which contributes to poverty reduction and better health for a section of
the worlds peoples but can equally cause job losses and deepen poverty

including ill-health in another part of the world. Almost all global public health institutions are affected by trade policies be they bilateral, plurilateral or multilateral trade agreements.

The World Health Organization in the 21st Century and beyond needs to encourage Member States to consider negotiating trade agreements with an outcome beneficial to public health, research, innovation and development. International trade remains the engine for inclusive economic growth and poverty reduction, and contributes to sustainable development.

The World Trade Organization provides the best platform for negotiating new multilateral trade agreements with potential for win-win outcomes and best prospects of protecting public health and contributing to improved health care for the worlds peoples. This is based to a large extent on personal knowledge and experience having had the honor and privilege to serve as Ambassador to the World Trade Organization, a member of the World Trade Organization Green Room, Coordinator of the African Group to the World Trade Organization, Chairman of the World Trade Organization Council for Trade in Goods and President of UNCTAD Trade and Investment Commission.

Chapter 10. Conclusion

In conclusion, there is adequate evidence that the overall health status
of the worlds peoples is not improving as was expected. There is need
for additional funding for research to find out why maternal mortality
rate, neonatal mortality rate and under-five mortality rate are off-track
and in the meantime increase funding to scale-up implementation of
interventions already proven to work in all settings. Research should
guide implementation of new activities towards achieving the
sustainable development goals. Strengthening the WHO Country Office
to provide quality technical assistance to States in need to develop or
review national health policies is necessary in order to mobilize
additional domestic and international resources.

Revitalizing managing relations between the World Health Organization
and the United Nations, UN Specialized agencies, International
Organizations, scientific and professional groups including non-State
actors is a critical success factor for effective and efficient global
leadership in health care in the 21st Century and beyond.

Part 2 of Health of Nation publication series shall discuss The Triad
Strategy, considered a new energy to power better health outcomes for
the worlds peoples in the 21st Century Plus.

Explanatory Notes on Introducing the Health of Nation

1. Maternal Mortality Ratio MMR is the number of maternal deaths per 100,000 live births. Based on information from the World Health organization, the number of women dying due to complications during pregnancy and childbirth decreased by 44% from an estimated 532 000 in 1990 to 303 000 in 2015. The progress is notable, but the annual rate of decline is less than half of what is needed to achieve the Millennium Development Goal (MDG) target of reducing the maternal mortality ratio by 75% between 1990 and 2015, which would require an annual decline of 5.5%. The 44% decline since 1990 translates into an average annual decline of just 2.3%. Between 1990 and 2000, the global maternal mortality ratio decreased by 1.2% per year, while from 2000 to 2015 progress accelerated to a 3.0% decline per year.

2. Neonatal Mortality Rate NMR is the number of neonatal deaths (deaths within 28 days of life) per 1000 live births. Based on the report from the World Health Organization, the neonatal mortality rate fell from 36 deaths per 1,000 live births in 1990 to 19 in 2015, and the number of neonatal deaths declined from 5.1 million to 2.7 million.

3. Infant Mortality Rate IMR is the number of infant deaths (child deaths within one year of life) per 1000 live births. Globally, infant mortality rate was 63 in 1990 got reduced to 32.

4. Under-five mortality rate U5MR is the number of child deaths under the age of five years per 1000 live births. Based on information from the World Health Organization since1990, the global under-five mortality rate dropped by 53 percent, from 91 deaths per 1,000 live births in 1990 to 43 in 2015.

5. The United Nations or UN is an Organization of 194 sovereign states or countries with its Headquarters in New York City and Offices at Geneva - UNOG, Vienna - UNOV and Nairobi - UNON. The UN principal organs are the General Assembly, Security Council, The Economic and Social Council - ECOSOC, The Secretariat headed by the UN Secretary-General, The International Court of Justice - ICJ and The Trusteeship Council.

6. The UN was established on 24 October 1945 when the UN Charter, which is an International Treaty was ratified. The name coined by US President Frankline D Roosevelt was first used in the "Declaration by United Nations" on first January 1942 during the Second World War when 26 nations pledged their governments to continue fighting against the Axis powers. The forerunner of the United Nations was the League of Nations, an organization established in 1919 under the Treaty of Versailles to promote international cooperation and to achieve peace and security, expired when it failed to prevent the Second World War.

7. In 1945 representatives of 50 countries met in San Francisco at the United Nations Conference on International Organization to draw up the United Nations Charter, which was signed on 26 June 1945 and ratified by China, France, the Soviet Union, the United Kingdom, the United States of America and a majority of other signatories on 24 October 1945. October 24 is observed as the United Nations Day. The draft UN charter was developed by the representatives of China, the Soviet Union, the United Kingdom and the United States at Dumbarton Oaks, United States, from August to October 1944. Poland though not represented at the Conference signed the UN Charter later and became one of the original 51 member states.

8. The purposes of UN is to maintain international peace and security; to develop friendly relations among nations based on the respect for the principle of equal rights and self-determination of peoples; to cooperate in solving international economic, social, cultural, and humanitarian problems and in promoting respect for human rights and fundamental freedoms; to be a Centre for harmonizing the actions of nations in attaining these common ends.

9. The UN acts in accordance with the principles that it is based on the sovereign equality of all its members; all members are to fulfill in good faith their charter obligations; they are to settle their international disputes by peaceful means and without endangering international peace and security and justice; they are to refrain from the threat or use of force against any other state; they are to give the United Nations every assistance in any action it takes in accordance with the Charter; nothing in the Charter is to authorize the United Nations to intervene in matters which are essentially within the domestic jurisdiction of any state.

10. The General Assembly consists of all the 194 members of the UN. It receives and considers reports from other organs of the UN, elects 10 non-permanent members of the Security Council and members of ECOSOC, ICJ and appoints the UNSG. The five permanent members P5 of the Security Council each with veto powers are China, France, Russia, United Kingdom and United States of America.

11. The Security Council is responsible for the maintenance of international peace and security by pacific settlement of disputes and action with respect to threats to the peace, breaches of the peace, and acts of aggression. It has P5 and 10 non-permanent members.

12. The Trusteeship Council made up of P5, completed its work on November 1 1994, and as such no longer meets, no longer exists since 2005. It was responsible for the administration and supervision of territories under colonization. Decolonization led to new 80 States coming into existence since 1945. Palau, an Island group in the Pacific was the last trust territory, and became a member of the UN on December 15, 1994.

13. The Economic and Social Council is responsible for promoting higher standards of living, full employment and conditions of economic and social progress and development; promoting solutions to international economic, social, health and related problems, and international cultural and education cooperation; promoting universal respect for, and observance of, rights and fundamental freedoms for all, without distinction as to race, sex, language or religion. It coordinates the work of United Nations Specialized agencies, UN Commissions, regional economic commissions for Africa, Asia and the Pacific, Europe, Latin America and Western Asia among others. It consults with academics, business sector representatives, and non-governmental organizations.

14. UN programs and funds include UN Children's Fund UNICEF; UN Development Programme UNDP; Office of the United Nations High Commissioner for Refugees UNHCR; United Nations Environmental Programme UNEP; UN Human Settlement Programme UN-HABITAT; World Food Programme WFP; UNAIDS; United Nations Conference on Trade and Development UNCTAD among others.

15. UN specialized agencies include International Labour Organization ILO; Food and Agriculture Organization of the United Nations FAO; United Nations Educational, Scientific and Cultural Organization UNESCO; World Health Organization WHO, The World Bank, International Monetary Fund IMF; International Telecommunications Union ITU, Universal Postal Union UPU, World Meteorological Organization WMO, World Intellectual Property Organization WIPO, United Nations Industrial Development Organization UNIDO among others.

16. The Office of the High Commissioner for Human Rights - OHCHR is the focal point for all human rights activities of the United Nations, acts as the secretariat for the meetings of the United Nations human rights bodies.

17. Human Rights Council HRC is a subsidiary body of the General Assembly responsible for promoting universal respect for the protection of all human rights and fundamental freedoms for all, without distinction of any kind and in a fair and equal manner. It is mandated to consider violations of human rights, including gross and systemic violations, and to make recommendations. The Council is also expected to promote the effective coordination and mainstreaming of human rights within the UN system.

18. The UN Treaty Bodies include Committee Against Torture CAT; Subcommittee on Prevention of Torture SPT; Committee on Elimination of Discrimination against Women CEDAW; Committee on Economic, Social, and Cultural Rights CESCR; Committee on the Elimination of Racial Discrimination CERD, Committee on the Rights of the Child CRC; Committee on the Protection of the Rights of All Migrant Workers and Members of Their Families CMW; Committee on the Rights of Persons with Disabilities CRPD, Human Rights Committee. The Universal Declaration of Human Rights is all about rights.

19. Member States of the United Nations who have agreed with its principles by signing and ratifying two international covenants, one addressing civil and political rights and the other economic, social, and cultural rights are legally bound. The Universal Declaration of Human Rights together with the International Covenant on Civil and Political Rights and the International Covenant on Economic, Social, Cultural Rights constitute the International Bill of Human Rights.

20. The World Health Organization highest governing body is the World Health Assembly WHA composed of 194 member states and meets annually. Its policies and decisions are given effect by the Executive Board composed of 34 government appointed health experts meeting twice a year. The Secretariat is headed by the Director-General appointed by WHA. WHA supervises the finances of the organization and is responsible for making WHO policies.

21. Pan American Health Organization - PAHO is WHO Regional Office for the Americas (AMRO) since 24 May 1949, has 35 Member States, Regional Office in Washington DC USA;

22. The other five WHO Regional Offices are the WHO African Region - AFRO 47 Member States, Regional Office in Brazzaville, Congo;

23. WHO South-East Asia Region SEARO 11 Member States, Regional Office in New Delhi India;

24. WHO European Region EURO 53 Member States, Regional Office in Copenhagen, Denmark;

25. WHO Eastern Mediterranean Region EMRO, 21 Member States, Regional Office in Cairo, Egypt;

26. WHO Western Pacific Region - WPRO 27 Member States, Regional Office in Manila Philippines.

27. The WHO Constitution was adopted by the International Health Conference held in New York from 19 June to 22 July 1946, signed on 22 July 1946 by the representatives of 61 States and entered into force on 7 April 1948. The first World Health Assembly was convened in Geneva in July 1948.

28. WHO has its roots on potential global impact of outbreaks on people and trade. Its establishment was preceded by seven international sanitary conferences in the 19th Century, Office of the International D'hygiene Publique in 1907, which cooperated closely with the Pan-American Sanitary Organization. The fist International convention on cholera was adopted in 1882 during the Seventh international sanitary conference.

29. The UN Secretariat is headed by the Secretary-General. It is composed of the Executive Office of the UNSG, Office of Internal Oversight Services, Office of Legal Affairs, Department of Political Affairs, Office of Disarmament Affairs, Department of Peacekeeping Operations, Department of Field Support, Office for Coordination of Humanitarian Affairs, Department for General Assembly and Conference Management, Department of Economic and Social Affairs, Department of Public Information, Department of Management, UN Ombudsman and Mediation Services and United Nations International Strategy for Disaster Reduction Secretariat.

30. The International Court of Justice principal function is to decide on, in accordance with international law, cases that are submitted to it by states. It gives advisory opinions to the General Assembly Security Council and other organs of the UN and specialized agencies when authorized by the General Assembly.

31. The GAVI Alliance is a partnership of public and private sector to improve child health in the poorest countries by extending the reach and quality of immunization coverage within strengthened health services. It has a Board which includes UNICEF, WHO, non-State actors, donor and implementing country governments, vaccine industry representatives, the Bill and Melinda Gates Foundation among others. The GAVI Fund is administered by a Secretariat headed by the Executive Director.

32. The World Trade Organization WTO; The Conference on Disarmament CD are not United Nations bodies but are in special relationship with The UN.

33. The World Trade Organization WTO, established on 1 January 1995 is an international organization in special relations with the United Nations helping trade to flow smoothly, freely, fairly and predictably by managing trade agreements, acting as a forum for trade negotiations, settling trade disputes, reviewing national trade policies, assisting developing countries in trade policy issues and cooperating with other international organizations.

34. In joint technical cooperation with UN Conference on Trade and Development UNCTAD, they established The International Trade Centre ITC in order to strengthen the international competitiveness of enterprises, develop the capacity of trade service providers to support businesses and support policy-makers in integrating the business sector into the global economy. The ITC was created in 1994 through a decision of the UN General Assembly on Tariff and Trade - GATT Contracting Parties. In 1968, UNCTAD joined GATT as a co-sponsor of the ITC. In 1974 ITC legal status was confirmed by The UN General Assembly as a joint subsidiary organ of GATT and the UN, with The UN acting through UNCTAD.

35. GATT was the precursor to the World Trade Organization.

36. The Conference on Disarmament CD, established in 1979 is a multilateral disarmament negotiating forum of the international community responsible for all multilateral arms control and disarmament problems. It succeeded the 1960 Ten-Nation Committee on Disarmament, the 1962-68 Eighteen-Nation Committee on Disarmament and the 1969-78 Conference of the Committee on Disarmament. The CD has a special relationship with the United Nations. It adopts its own Rules of Procedure and its own agenda, taking into account the recommendations of the General Assembly and the proposals of its Members.

37. The Conference on Disarmament puts greater focus on Nuclear weapons in all aspects; chemical weapons; other weapons of mass destruction; conventional weapons; reduction of military budgets; reduction of armed forces; disarmament and development; disarmament and international security; collateral measures, confidence-building measures and effective verification methods in relation to appropriate disarmament measures, acceptable to all parties concerned; comprehensive programme of disarmament leading to general and complete disarmament under effective international control.

38. The International Telecommunications Union ITU, was founded in 1865 as the International Telegraph Union. It is now a specialized agency of the UN. The 1932 Madrid Plenipotentiary Conference decided on the current name which came into force from 1 January 1934. ITU brings together governments and industry to coordinate

the establishment and operation of global telecommunications networks and services.

39. The Universal Postal Union was established in 1874 by the Bern Treaty. It a specialized agency of the United Nations since 1948. UPU aims to secure the Organization and improvement of postal services, promote the development of international collaboration and undertake, as far as possible, technical assistance in postal matters requested by member states who constitute a single postal territory.

40. In 1899, the first International Peace Conference was held in The Hague to elaborate instruments of settling crises peacefully, preventing wars and codifying rules of warfare. It adopted the convention for the Pacific Settlement of International Disputes and established the Permanent Court of Arbitration, which began work in 1902.

41. The International Labour Organizations ILO was founded in 1919 under the Treaty of Versailles, as an affiliated agency of the League of Nations. ILO became the first specialized agency of the United Nations in 1946. It is the only 'tripartite ' UN agency whose members include governments, employers and workers shaping its policies and programmes. ILO aims to promote rights at work; encourage decent employment opportunities; enhance social protection; strengthen dialogue in handling work-related issues.

42. WHO Regional Groupings. There are six WHO Region Groupings of Member States. They are:

43. WHO African Region: Algeria, Angola, Benin, Botswana, Burkina Faso, Burundi, Cabo Verde, Cameroon, Central African Republic, Chad, Comoros, Congo, C te d'Ivoire, Democratic Republic of the Congo, Equatorial Guinea, Eritrea, Ethiopia, Gabon, Gambia, Ghana, Guinea, Guinea-Bissau, Kenya, Lesotho, Liberia, Madagascar, Malawi, Mali, Mauritania, Mauritius, Mozambique, Namibia, Niger, Nigeria, Rwanda, Sao Tome and Principe, Senegal, Seychelles, Sierra Leone, South Africa, South Sudan, Swaziland, Togo, Uganda, United Republic of Tanzania, Zambia, Zimbabwe.

44. WHO Region of the Americas: Antigua and Barbuda, Argentina, Bahamas, Barbados, Belize, Bolivia (Plurinational State of), Brazil, Canada, Chile, Colombia, Costa Rica, Cuba, Dominica, Dominican Republic, Ecuador, El Salvador, Grenada, Guatemala, Guyana, Haiti, Honduras, Jamaica, Mexico, Nicaragua, Panama, Paraguay, Peru, Saint Kitts and Nevis, Saint Lucia, Saint Vincent and the Grenadines, Suriname, Trinidad and Tobago, United States of America, Uruguay, Venezuela (Bolivarian Republic of).

45. WHO South-East Asia Region: Bangladesh, Bhutan, Democratic People's Republic of Korea, India, Indonesia, Maldives, Myanmar, Nepal, Sri Lanka, Thailand, Timor-Leste.

46. WHO European Region: Albania, Andorra, Armenia, Austria, Azerbaijan, Belarus, Belgium, Bosnia and Herzegovina, Bulgaria, Croatia, Cyprus, Czech Republic, Denmark, Estonia, Finland, France, Georgia, Germany, Greece, Hungary, Iceland, Ireland, Israel, Italy, Kazakhstan, Kyrgyzstan, Latvia, Lithuania, Luxembourg, Malta, Monaco, Montenegro, Netherlands, Norway, Poland, Portugal, Republic of Moldova, Romania, Russian Federation, San Marino, Serbia, Slovakia, Slovenia, Spain, Sweden, Switzerland, Tajikistan, The former Yugoslav Republic of Macedonia, Turkey, Turkmenistan, Ukraine, United Kingdom, Uzbekistan.

47. WHO Eastern Mediterranean Region: Afghanistan, Bahrain, Djibouti, Egypt, Iran (Islamic Republic of), Iraq, Jordan, Kuwait, Lebanon, Libya, Morocco, Oman, Pakistan, Qatar, Saudi Arabia, Somalia, Sudan, Syrian Arab Republic, Tunisia, United Arab Emirates, Yemen.

48. WHO Western Pacific Region: Australia, Brunei Darussalam, Cambodia, China, Cook Islands, Fiji, Japan, Kiribati, Lao People's Democratic Republic, Malaysia, Marshall Islands, Micronesia (Federated States of), Mongolia, Nauru, New Zealand, Niue, Palau, Papua New Guinea, Philippines, Republic of Korea, Samoa, Singapore, Solomon Islands, Tonga, Tuvalu, Vanuatu, Vietnam.

Chapter

Appendix B

Universal Declaration of Human Rights

Preamble

Whereas recognition of the inherent dignity and of the equal and inalienable rights of all members of the human family is the foundation of freedom, justice and peace in the world,

Whereas disregard and contempt for human rights have resulted in barbarous acts which have outraged the conscience of mankind, and the advent of a world in which human beings shall enjoy freedom of speech and belief and freedom from fear and want has been proclaimed as the highest aspiration of the common people,

Whereas it is essential, if man is not to be compelled to have recourse, as a last resort, to rebellion against tyranny and oppression, that human rights should be protected by the rule of law,

Whereas it is essential to promote the development of friendly relations between nations,

Whereas the peoples of the United Nations have in the Charter reaffirmed their faith in fundamental human rights, in the dignity and worth of the human person and in the equal rights of men and women and have determined to promote social progress and better standards of life in larger freedom,

Whereas Member States have pledged themselves to achieve, in cooperation with the United Nations, the promotion of universal respect for and observance of human rights and fundamental freedoms,

Whereas a common understanding of these rights and freedoms is of the greatest importance for the full realization of this pledge,

Now, therefore,

The General Assembly,

Proclaims this Universal Declaration of Human Rights as a common standard of achievement for all peoples and all nations, to the end that every individual and every organ of society, keeping this Declaration constantly in mind, shall strive by

teaching and education to promote respect for these rights and freedoms and by progressive measures, national and international, to secure their universal and effective recognition and observance, both among the peoples of Member States themselves and among the peoples of territories under their jurisdiction.

Article I

All human beings are born free and equal in dignity and rights. They are endowed with reason and conscience and should act towards one another in a spirit of brotherhood.

Article 2

Everyone is entitled to all the rights and freedoms set forth in this Declaration, without distinction of any kind, such as race, colour, sex, language, religion, political or other opinion, national or social origin, property, birth or other status. Furthermore, no distinction shall be made on the basis of the political, jurisdictional or international status of the country or territory to which a person belongs, whether it be independent, trust, non-self-governing or under any other limitation of sovereignty.

Article 3

Everyone has the right to life, liberty and security of person.

Article 4

No one shall be held in slavery or servitude; slavery and the slave trade shall be prohibited in all their forms.

Article 5

No one shall be subjected to torture or to cruel, inhuman or degrading treatment or punishment.

Article 6

Everyone has the right to recognition everywhere as a person before the law. Article 7

All are equal before the law and are entitled without any discrimination to equal protection of the law. All are entitled to equal protection against any discrimination in violation of this Declaration and against any incitement to such discrimination.

Article 8

Everyone has the right to an effective remedy by the competent national tribunals for acts violating the fundamental rights granted him by the constitution or by law.

Article 9

No one shall be subjected to arbitrary arrest, detention or exile. Article 10

Everyone is entitled in full equality to a fair and public hearing by an independent and impartial tribunal, in the determination of his rights and obligations and of any criminal charge against him.

Article 11

1. Everyonechargedwithapenaloffencehastherighttobepresumed innocent until proved guilty according to law in a public trial at which he has had all the guarantees necessary for his defence.

2. Nooneshallbeheldguiltyofanypenaloffenceonaccountofanyactor omission which did not constitute a penal offence, under national or international law, at the time when it was committed. Nor shall a heavier penalty be imposed than the one that was applicable at the time the penal offence was committed.

Article 12

No one shall be subjected to arbitrary interference with his privacy, family, home or correspondence, nor to attacks upon his honour and reputation. Everyone has the right to the protection of the law against such interference or attacks.

Article 13

1. Everyonehastherighttofreedomofmovementandresidencewithinthe borders of each State.

2. Everyone has the right to leave any country, including his own, and to return to his country.

Article 14

1. Everyone has the right to seek and to enjoy in other countries asylum from persecution.

2. Thisrightmaynotbeinvokedinthecaseofprosecutionsgenuinely arising from non-political crimes or from acts contrary to the purposes and principles of the United Nations.

Article 15

1. Everyonehastherighttoanationality.

2. No one shall be arbitrarily deprived of his nationality nor denied the right to change his nationality.

Article 16

1. Men and women of full age, without any limitation due to race, nationality or religion, have the right to marry and to found a family. They are entitled to equal rights as to marriage, during marriage and at its dissolution.

2. Marriageshallbeenteredintoonlywiththefreeandfullconsentofthe intending spouses.

3. The family is the natural and fundamental group unit of society and is entitled to protection by society and the State.

Article 17

1. Everyonehastherighttoownpropertyaloneaswellasinassociationwith others.

2. Nooneshallbearbitrarilydeprivedofhisproperty.

Article 18

Everyone has the right to freedom of thought, conscience and religion; this right includes freedom to change his religion or belief, and freedom, either alone or in community with others and in public or private, to manifest his religion or belief in teaching, practice, worship and observance.

Article 19

Everyone has the right to freedom of opinion and expression; this right includes freedom to hold opinions without interference and to seek, receive and impart information and ideas through any media and regardless of frontiers.

Article 20

1. Everyonehastherighttofreedomofpeacefulassemblyandassociation. 2. Noonemaybecompelledtobelongtoanassociation.

Article 21

Everyonehastherighttotakepartinthegovernmentofhiscountry, directly or through freely chosen representatives.

2. Everyonehastherighttoequalaccesstopublicserviceinhiscountry.

3. Thewillofthepeopleshallbethebasisoftheauthorityofgovernment;

this will shall be expressed in periodic and genuine elections which shall be by universal and equal suffrage and shall be held by secret vote or by equivalent free voting procedures.

Article 22

Everyone, as a member of society, has the right to social security and is entitled to realization, through national effort and international co-operation and in accordance with the organization and resources of each State, of the economic, social and cultural rights indispensable for his dignity and the free development of his personality.

Article 23

1. Everyone has the right to work, to free choice of employment, to just and favourable conditions of work and to protection against unemployment.

2. Everyone, without any discrimination, has the right to equal pay for equal work.

3. Everyonewhoworkshastherighttojustandfavourableremuneration ensuring for himself and his family an existence worthy of human dignity, and supplemented, if necessary, by other means of social protection.

4. Everyone has the right to form and to join trade unions for the protection of his interests.

Article 24

Everyone has the right to rest and leisure, including reasonable limitation of working hours and periodic holidays with pay.

Article 25

1. Everyonehastherighttoastandardoflivingadequateforthehealthand well-being of himself and of his family, including food, clothing, housing and medical care and necessary social services, and the right to security in the event of unemployment, sickness, disability, widowhood, old age or other lack of livelihood in circumstances beyond his control.

2. Motherhoodandchildhoodareentitledtospecialcareandassistance.All children, whether born in or out of wedlock, shall enjoy the same social protection.

Article 26

1. Everyone has the right to education. Education shall be free, at least in the elementary and fundamental stages. Elementary education shall be compulsory. Technical and professional education shall be made generally available and higher education shall be equally accessible to all on the basis of merit.

2. Educationshallbedirectedtothefulldevelopmentofthehuman personality and to the strengthening of respect for human rights and fundamental freedoms. It shall promote understanding, tolerance and friendship among all nations, racial or religious groups, and shall further the activities of the United Nations for the maintenance of peace.

3. Parents have a prior right to choose the kind of education that shall be given to their children.

Article 27

1. Everyonehastherightfreelytoparticipateintheculturallifeofthe community, to enjoy the arts and to share in scientific advancement and its benefits.

2. Everyonehastherighttotheprotectionofthemoralandmaterialinterests resulting from any scientific, literary or artistic production of which he is the author.

Article 28

Everyone is entitled to a social and international order in which the rights and freedoms set forth in this Declaration can be fully realized.

Article 29

1. Everyonehasdutiestothecommunityinwhichalonethefreeandfull development of his personality is possible.

2. In the exercise of his rights and freedoms, everyone shall be subject only to such limitations as are determined by law solely for the purpose of securing due recognition and respect for the rights and freedoms of

others and of meeting the just requirements of morality, public order and the general welfare in a democratic society.

3. Theserightsandfreedomsmayinnocasebeexercisedcontrarytothe purposes and principles of the United Nations.

Article 30

Nothing in this Declaration may be interpreted as implying for any State, group or person any right to engage in any activity or to perform any act aimed at the destruction of any of the rights and freedoms set forth herein.

Appendix C

Sustainable Development Goals 2016 - 2030

Goal 1. End poverty in all its forms everywhere

Goal 2. End hunger, achieve food security and improved nutrition and promote sustainable agriculture

Goal 3. Ensure healthy lives and promote well-being for all at all ages

Goal 4. Ensure inclusive and equitable quality education and promote lifelong learning opportunities for all

Goal 5. Achieve gender equality and empower all women and girls

Goal 6. Ensure availability and sustainable management of water and sanitation for all

Goal 7. Ensure access to affordable, reliable, sustainable and modern energy for all

Goal 8. Promote sustained, inclusive and sustainable economic growth, full and productive employment and decent work for all

Goal 9. Build resilient infrastructure, promote inclusive and sustainable industrialization and foster innovation

Goal 10. Reduce inequality within and among countries

Goal 11. Make cities and human settlements inclusive, safe, resilient and sustainable

Goal 12. Ensure sustainable consumption and production patterns

Goal 13. Take urgent action to combat climate change and its impacts*

Goal 14. Conserve and sustainably use the oceans, seas and marine resources for sustainable development

Goal 15. Protect, restore and promote sustainable use of terrestrial ecosystems, sustainably manage forests, combat desertification, and halt and reverse land degradation and halt biodiversity loss

Goal 16. Promote peaceful and inclusive societies for sustainable development, provide access to justice for all and build effective, accountable and inclusive institutions at all levels

Goal 17. Strengthen the means of implementation and revitalize the Global Partnership for Sustainable Development

* Acknowledging that the United Nations Framework Convention on Climate Change is the primary international, intergovernmental forum for negotiating the global response to climate change.

Appendix D

Millennium Development Goals 1990 - 2015

Goal 1: Eradicate polio Extreme Hunger and Poverty

Target 1. Halve, between 1990 and 2015, the proportion of people whose income is less than $1 a day

Indicators

1. Proportion of population below $1 (1993 PPP) per day (World Bank) a*

2. Poverty gap ratio [incidence x depth of poverty] (World Bank)

3. Share of poorest quintile in national consumption (World Bank)

Target 2. Halve, between 1990 and 2015, the proportion of people who suffer from hunger

Indicators

4. Prevalence of underweight children under five years of age (UNICEF-WHO)

5. Proportion of population below minimum level of dietary energy consumption (FAO)

Goal 2: Achieve Universal Primary Education

Target 3. Ensure that, by 2015, children everywhere, boys and girls alike, will be able to complete a full course of primary schooling

Indicators

6. Net enrolment ratio in primary education (UNESCO)

7. Proportion of pupils starting grade 1 who reach grade 5 (UNESCO) b*

8. Literacy rate of 15-24 year-olds (UNESCO)

Goal 3: Promote Gender Equality and Empower Women

Target 4. Eliminate gender disparity in primary and secondary education, preferably by 2005, and in all levels of education no later than 2015

Indicators

9. Ratio of girls to boys in primary, secondary and tertiary education (UNESCO)

10. Ratio of literate women to men, 15-24 years old (UNESCO)

11. Share of women in wage employment in the non-agricultural sector (ILO)

12. Proportion of seats held by women in national parliament (IPU)

Goal 4: Reduce Child Mortality

Target 5. Reduce by two-thirds, between 1990 and 2015, the under-five mortality rate

Indicators

13. Under-five mortality rate (UNICEF-WHO)

14. Infant mortality rate (UNICEF-WHO)

15. Proportion of 1 year-old children immunized against measles (UNICEF-WHO)

Goal 4: Reduce Child Mortality

Target 5. Reduce by two-thirds, between 1990 and 2015, the under-five mortality rate

Indicators

13. Under-five mortality rate (UNICEF-WHO)

14. Infant mortality rate (UNICEF-WHO)

15. Proportion of 1 year-old children immunized against measles (UNICEF-WHO)

Goal 5: Improve Maternal Health

Target 6. Reduce by three-quarters, between 1990 and 2015, the maternal mortality ratio

Indicators

16. Maternal mortality ratio (UNICEF-WHO)

17. Proportion of births attended by skilled health personnel (UNICEF-WHO)

Goal 6: Combat HIV/AIDS, Malaria and other diseases

Target 7. Have halted by 2015 and begun to reverse the spread of HIV/AIDS

Indicators

18. HIV prevalence among pregnant women aged 15-24 years (UNAIDS-WHO-UNICEF)

19. Condom use rate of the contraceptive prevalence rate (UN Population Division) c*

19a. Condom use at last high-risk sex (UNICEF-WHO)

19b. Percentage of population aged 15-24 years with comprehensive correct knowledge of HIV/AIDS (UNICEF-WHO) d*

19c. Contraceptive prevalence rate (UN Population Division)

20. Ratio of school attendance of orphans to school attendance of non-orphans aged 10-14 years (UNICEF-UNAIDS-WHO)

Target 8. Have halted by 2015 and begun to reverse the incidence of malaria and other major diseases

Indicators

21. Prevalence and death rates associated with malaria (WHO)

22. Proportion of population in malaria-risk areas using effective malaria prevention and treatment measures (UNICEF-WHO) e*

23. Prevalence and death rates associated with tuberculosis (WHO)

24. Proportion of tuberculosis cases detected and cured under DOTS (internationally recommended TB control strategy) (WHO)

Goal 7: Ensure Environmental Sustainability

Target 9. Integrate the principles of sustainable development into country policies and programs and reverse the loss of environmental resources

Indicators

25. Proportion of land area covered by forest (FAO)

26. Ratio of area protected to maintain biological diversity to surface area (UNEP-WCMC)

27. Energy use (kg oil equivalent) per $1 GDP (PPP) (IEA, World Bank)

28. Carbon dioxide emissions per capita (UNFCCC, UNSD) and consumption of ozone-depleting CFCs (ODP tons) (UNEP-Ozone Secretariat)

29. Proportion of population using solid fuels (WHO)

Target 10. Halve, by 2015, the proportion of people without sustainable access to safe drinking water and basic sanitation

Indicators

30. Proportion of population with sustainable access to an improved water source, urban and rural (UNICEF-WHO)

31. Proportion of population with access to improved sanitation, urban and rural (UNICEF-WHO)

Target 11. Have achieved by 2020 a significant improvement in the lives of at least 100 million slum dwellers

Indicators

32. Proportion of households with access to secure tenure (UN-HABITAT)

Goal 8: Develop a Global Partnership for Development

Target 12. Develop further an open, rule-based, predictable, nondiscriminatory trading and financial system (includes a commitment to good governance, development, and poverty reduction? both nationally and internationally)

Target 13. Address the special needs of the Least Developed Countries (includes tariff- and quota-free access for Least Developed Countries? exports, enhanced program of debt relief for heavily indebted poor countries [HIPCs] and cancellation of official bilateral debt, and more generous official development assistance for countries committed to poverty reduction)

Target 14. Address the special needs of landlocked developing countries and small island developing states (through the Program of Action for the Sustainable Development of Small Island Developing States and 22nd General Assembly provisions)

Target 15. Deal comprehensively with the debt problems of developing countries through national and international measures in order to make debt sustainable in the long term

Indicators

Official development assistance (ODA)

33. Net ODA, total and to LDCs, as percentage of OECD/Development Assistance Committee (DAC) donors' gross national income (GNI)(OECD)

34. Proportion of total bilateral, sector-allocable ODA of OECD/DAC donors to basic social services (basic education, primary health care, nutrition, safe water and sanitation) (OECD)

35. Proportion of bilateral ODA of OECD/DAC donors that is untied (OECD)

36. ODA received in landlocked developing countries as a proportion of their GNIs (OECD)

37. ODA received in small island developing States as proportion of their GNIs (OECD)

Market access

38. Proportion of total developed country imports (by value and excluding arms) from developing countries and from LDCs, admitted free of duty (UNCTAD, WTO, WB)

39. Average tariffs imposed by developed countries on agricultural products and textiles and clothing from developing countries (UNCTAD, WTO, WB)

40. Agricultural support estimate for OECD countries as percentage of their GDP (OECD)

41. Proportion of ODA provided to help build trade capacity (OECD, WTO)

Debt sustainability

42. Total number of countries that have reached their Heavily Indebted Poor Countries Initiative (HIPC) decision points and number that have reached their HIPC completion points (cumulative) (IMF - World Bank)

43. Debt relief committed under HIPC initiative (IMF-World Bank)

44. Debt service as a percentage of exports of goods and services (IMF-World Bank)

Some of the indicators listed below are monitored separately for the least developed countries, Africa, landlocked developing countries, and small island developing states

Target 16. In cooperation with developing countries, develop and implement strategies for decent and productive work for youth

Indicators

45. Unemployment rate of young people aged 15-24 years, each sex and total (ILO) f*

Target 17. In cooperation with pharmaceutical companies, provide access to affordable essential drugs in developing countries

Indicators

46. Proportion of population with access to affordable essential drugs on a sustainable basis (WHO)

Target 18. In cooperation with the private sector, make available the benefits of new technologies, especially information and communications technologie

Indicators

47. Telephone lines and cellular subscribers per 100 population (ITU)

48. Personal computers in use per 100 population and Internet users per 100 population (ITU)